Und

Controlling the Irritable
B

Magdy El-Salhy
Jan Gunnar Hatlebakk
Trygve Hausken

Understanding and Controlling the Irritable Bowel

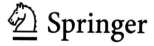 Springer

Magdy El-Salhy
Clinical Medicine
University of Bergen
Bergen, Norway

Jan Gunnar Hatlebakks
Clinical Medicine
University of Bergen
Bergen, Norway

Trygve Hausken
Clinical Medicine
University of Bergen
Bergen, Norway

ISBN 978-3-319-15641-5   ISBN 978-3-319-15642-2   (eBook)
DOI 10.1007/978-3-319-15642-2

Library of Congress Control Number: 2015937614

Springer Cham Heidelberg New York Dordrecht London
© Springer International Publishing Switzerland 2015

Printed on acid-free paper

Springer International Publishing AG Switzerland is part of Springer Science+Business Media (www.springer.com)

Preface

Irritable bowel syndrome (IBS) is a common disorder that affects up to one-fifth of the Western world. In addition to those who are diagnosed with IBS, there are many undiagnosed patients who ignore their symptoms and consider them simply to be a part of their everyday life. These individuals never visit healthcare centers or meet with a doctor in relation to their condition. The true number of individuals suffering from IBS is therefore much greater than that reported in the literature.

Despite undergoing several tests and examinations, and after repeated contact with their healthcare providers, many IBS sufferers are dissatisfied with their management and feel that they are either misunderstood or regarded as hypochondriacs or mentally ill. There is a widespread belief in society and among healthcare providers that IBS is unimportant since it is not a life-threatening disease. Furthermore, the consequences of suffering from IBS are often ignored; the considerable reduction in the patient's quality of life as a result of IBS, which may lead to social isolation, quitting work, and broken relationships, should not be underestimated.

Many IBS patients worry that their symptoms are either caused by a serious disease or that they will develop into a serious disease over time. Access to reliable information about IBS is important to both IBS patients and their healthcare providers. Some studies have shown that IBS patients who are not provided with support are able to correctly avoid some foodstuffs that can aggravate their symptoms, but they may replace them with items that are even worse. Several studies have shown that providing IBS-directed information to patients will improve their symptom and quality of life considerably.

We believe that information about IBS to both physicians and patients is important. In 2012 we wrote a book about IBS that was aimed at physicians, with a view to updating their knowledge base and informing them about the progress that has been made in our understanding of IBS and its management. The aims of the present book are to provide information directly to IBS patients, including providing them with strategies for controlling or managing the condition.

How to Read This Book

The aim of this book was to provide information about irritable bowel syndrome to enable patients suffering from this disorder to control it and to prevent it from interfering with their everyday activities. The intention was for this book to be easy to read and for the information it contains to be readily and quickly accessible. In order to achieve this, each chapter begins with a summary containing the most important points, and includes a large number of illustrations. Thus, the reader can obtain a quick overview by simply reading the summary of each chapter and going through the illustrations; chapters of interest can be read in more detail when more time is available.

Acknowledgements

The authors wish to thank Arnstein Mygland for his illustration of the figures in the first chapter, and figures in the appendix, Ingjerd Monsen Hjelmeland for the illustrations in Chaps. 2 and 3, and Tiril Hjelmeland for the photographs in Chap. 5.

Contents

About the Authors

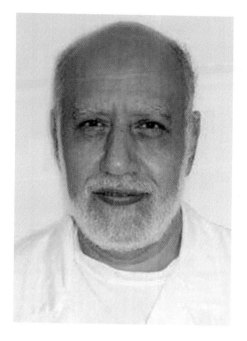

Magdy El-Salhy is Professor of Gastroenterology and Hepatology at the School of Medicine, University of Bergen, and is a consultant gastroenterologist at Stord Hospital, Norway. He completed his PhD (Medicine) in 1981 and his MD in 1989, both at Uppsala University, Sweden. Professor El-Salhy has 194 publications, which include original articles, invited reviews, book chapters, and books. His work has been cited in 3598 scientific articles, and he is on the editorial board of 8 international scientific journals. His research field for the last 40 years has been the neuroendocrine system of the gastrointestinal tract, from basic science to clinical applications. During the last 10 years he has focused his research on irritable bowel syndrome.

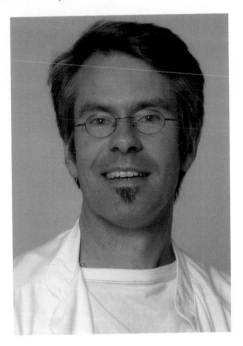

Jan Gunnar Hatlebakk is a consultant gastroenterologist at Haukeland University Hospital, Professor of Gastroenterology, Hepatology and Clinical Nutrition at University of Bergen Medical School, Norway, and head of the National Center for Functional Gastrointestinal Disorders. He was educated at the University of Bergen, achieving an MD in 1984 and a PhD in 1997. He completed his clinical training at Haukeland University Hospital and has performed postdoctoral research at The Graduate Hospital, Philadelphia (USA), and Université de Nantes (France). Professor Hatlebakk's research interests have included functional gastrointestinal disorders as well as gastroesophageal reflux and gastrointestinal motility disorders.

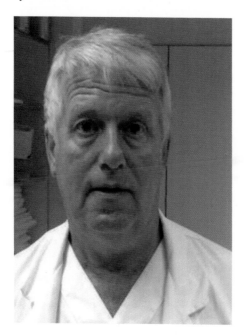

Trygve Hausken is Professor of Gastroenterology and Nutrition, and head of the gastroenterology section as well as a consultant gastroenterologist at Haukeland University Hospital, School of Medicine, University of Bergen, Norway. He completed his PhD (Medicine) in 1992 and has been a specialist in gastroenterology at Haukeland University Hospital since 1989. He has published 163 articles, including original papers, invited reviews, book chapters, and books. Professor Hausken's research fields have been functional gastrointestinal disorders, low-grade inflammation, gastrointestinal motility, and gastrointestinal ultrasonography, including nutritional imaging and 3D and 4D ultrasound, from basic science to clinical applications.

Chapter 1
Irritable Bowel Syndrome: What Is It?

Summary

- Irritable bowel syndrome (IBS) is a common gastrointestinal disorder that affects between 5 and 20 % of the Western world.
- IBS is characterized by abdominal discomfort or pain and changes in the frequency and appearance of the stool, with diarrhea or constipation, or a combination of the two, as well as abdominal distension.
- IBS considerably reduces the patient's quality of life, but does not develop into a serious disease or shorten the lifespan.
- Symptoms can occur in parts of the digestive system other than the large bowel, such as non-heart-related chest pain, stomachache, and gallstone-like attack.
- Some IBS patients suffer associated symptoms in other organs of the body, such as headache, fibromyalgia, chronic fatigue, depression and/or sleeping difficulties, and pain from the urogenital system.

M. El-Salhy et al., *Understanding and Controlling the Irritable Bowel*, DOI 10.1007/978-3-319-15642-2_1,
© Springer International Publishing Switzerland 2015

What Is Irritable Bowel Syndrome?

Irritable bowel syndrome (IBS) has been a recognized condition for thousands of years, since it is mentioned in ancient Egyptian papyri. In modern times this disorder has been discussed in the medical literature since Edson and colleagues reported on it in 1946. With the research methods of that time a medical explanation for the patient's symptoms could not be found. IBS is characterized by abdominal discomfort and/or pain and changes in the frequency and appearance of the stool, with diarrhea or constipation, or a combination of the two, as well as abdominal distension (Figs. 1.1, 1.2, 1.3, and 1.4). Some patients suffer from daily symptoms, while others report discontinuous symptoms at intervals of weeks or months. The intensity of the symptoms varies between patients from tolerable to severe, and the pain may be experienced as nagging, colicky, sharp, or dull. The symptoms can fluctuate in a patient over time, from mild or moderate symptoms at one particular time, to severe at another. Women usually experience severe symptoms during their menstruation period, and either mild or no symptoms at all during pregnancy.

IBS is a common disorder that reportedly affects 5–20 % of the Western world, with a female/male ratio of 2:1. About 20 % of the populations in Norway and Sweden suffer from IBS. Most (50–90 %) of IBS patients do not seek healthcare, instead ignoring their symptoms and regarding them as a normal part of their everyday life. Therefore, the true proportion of individuals suffering from IBS exceeds 20 % of the population. In Asia, where most of the people on Earth live, IBS affects 5–9 % of the population. Furthermore, IBS in Asia is not dominant in women, and the symptoms are different from those reported in the Western world. IBS patients in Asia complain mostly of abdominal distension and discomfort rather than abdominal pain, and they are not bothered by alterations in bowel habits. This difference in IBS between the West and Asia is attributed to differences in food intake (with the food habits of Asians preventing the developments

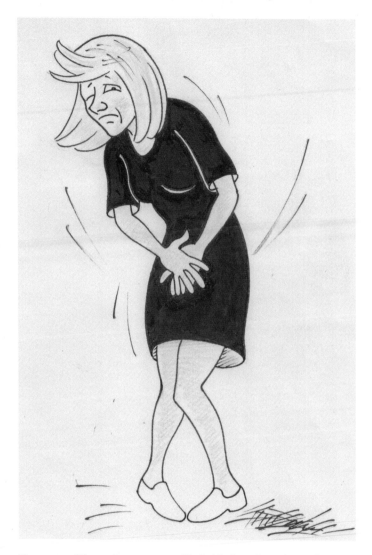

FIGURE 1.1 The main symptom of irritable bowel syndrome is recurrent abdominal pain or discomfort, which can be localized to one particular place or may move to different locations from time to time. When it occurs, the pain is mostly of a colic type

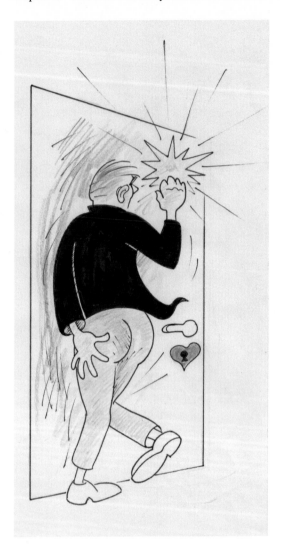

FIGURE 1.2 The second symptom of irritable bowel syndrome is periods of diarrhea, either alone or alternating with periods of constipation

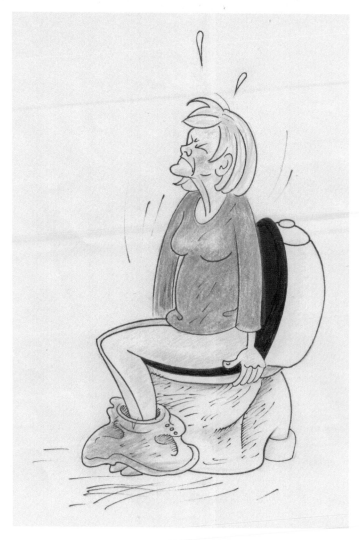

FIGURE 1.3 Constipation is the predominant symptom in about one-third of patients with irritable bowel syndrome

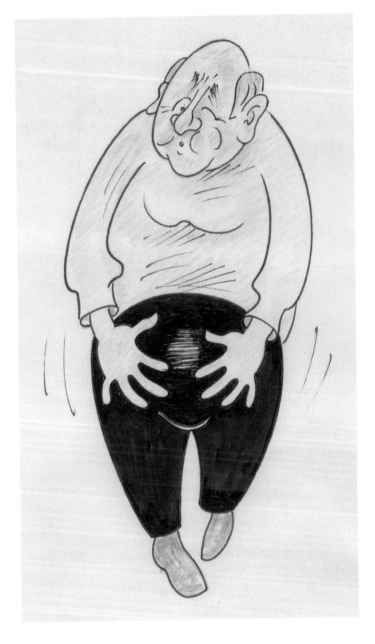

of IBS), differences in hygiene conditions (resulting in the development of immunological tolerance), and differences in the large-bowel bacteria (see Chap. 3). There are other factors that may contribute to the low prevalence of IBS in Asia. For example, it could be due to a cultural difference in healthcare-seeking behavior; it has been reported that Hispanics are less likely than non-Hispanics to seek healthcare for bowel complaints, and Hispanics are also more likely to self-medicate with folk remedies to maintain good bowel function. Furthermore, education and social status may play a role in the low rate of IBS in Asia.

IBS reduces the patient's quality of life considerably, to the same extent as major chronic diseases such as diabetes, heart failure, kidney failure, liver insufficiency, and other gastrointestinal diseases such as inflammatory bowel diseases. This negative change in quality of life may lead to social isolation, quitting work, and broken relationships. It has been reported that the average duration of sick leave from work for a patient with IBS is about 15 days per year in USA and 17 days in Norway. However, IBS is not known to be associated with the development of serious disease or excesses of deaths.

FIGURE 1.4 Abdominal distention occurs in patients with irritable bowel syndrome in addition to the symptoms mentioned in Figure. 1.1, 1.2 and 1.3

Other Symptoms Associated with IBS

Symptoms from Other Parts of the Digestive System in IBS Patients

Patients with IBS may have symptoms that originate from other parts of the digestive system. Although the reason for this is not completely understood, it seems that in some patients the disturbance of motility—the ability of the gastrointestinal tract to propel food through the digestive system, as described in the section entitled "The gastrointestinal tract and how it functions"—is not restricted to the large bowel, instead also affecting the esophagus, stomach, small bowel, and bile ducts. The following non-large bowel-related symptoms may occur: non-heart-related chest pain, stomach ache, and gallstone-like attacks.

Non-heart-Related Chest Pain

Reportedly 22–48 % of IBS patients experience episodes of pain in the middle of the chest (Fig. 1.5). Extensive investigation of the heart reveals a normal heart condition in these individuals. Intensive examination of the esophagus, including esophagogastroduodenoscopy, reveals normal findings. This symptom is believed to be the result of cramps in the muscles of the esophagus.

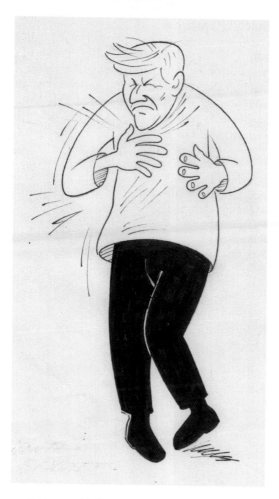

FIGURE 1.5 Patients with irritable bowel syndrome can suffer from other symptoms originating in other parts of the digestive tract, such as non-heart-related chest pain, which is probably caused by cramps in the esophagus

Stomachache (Gastritis)

Reportedly 7–42 % of IBS patients suffer periods of stomach ache, which doctors refer to as gastritis or dyspepsia (Fig. 1.6). Extensive investigation, including gastroscopy, does not reveal any abnormalities. The cause of this symptom is unknown, but it is probably cramps in the stomach and/or excessive gastric acid secretion.

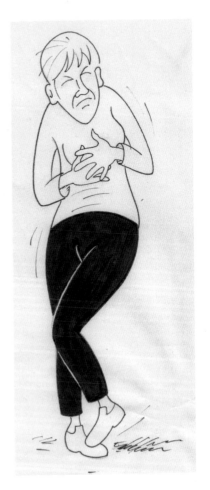

FIGURE 1.6 Stomachache is another symptom that originates from the stomach, and is probably caused by cramps of the stomach in patients with irritable bowel syndrome

Gallstone-Like Attack

A few patients suffer from periods of colicky pain in the upper right part of the abdomen (Fig. 1.7). The pain is just as intense as that experienced with gallstones, and occurs in the same location, but ultrasound examination in these patients reveals no gallstones. This condition is attributed to dysfunc-

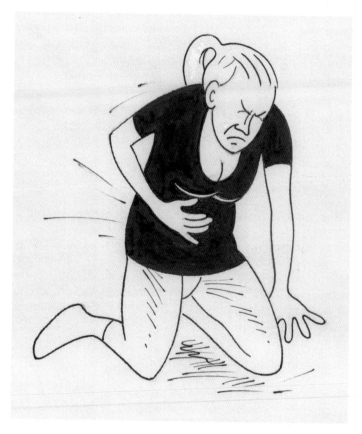

FIGURE 1.7 Some patients with irritable bowel syndrome are also affected by gallstone-like attacks, a symptom that is attributed to dysfunction of the coordination between the gallbladder and the muscle lining the bile duct

tion in the coordination between the gallbladder and the muscles lining the bile duct (sphincter of Oddi), and is thus described by doctors as sphincter of Oddi dyskinesia.

Symptoms from Parts of the Body Other Than the Digestive System in IBS Patients

In addition to their IBS symptoms, patients may also suffer from one or more of the following symptoms from other organs of the body: headache, fibromyalgia syndrome and chronic fatigue, depression and sleeping difficulties, and pain originating from the urinary and reproductive organs.

Headache

Reportedly 30–50 % of IBS patients suffer from headache, the cause of which is believed to be tension in the head and shoulder muscles (Fig. 1.8).

Fibromyalgia Syndrome and Chronic Fatigue

Some IBS patients suffer from fibromyalgia, which is diffuse muscle-related pain with sore points (Fig. 1.9), and chronic fatigue, which is fatigue that lasts for more than 6 months without any known medical reason (Fig. 1.10). The proportion of patients with IBS who suffer from these two symptoms is unknown, as is their cause.

Depression and Sleeping Difficulties

The reported proportion of IBS patients with depression differs between studies, but an association between IBS and depression and/or sleeping difficulties does exist (Figs. 1.11 and 1.12).

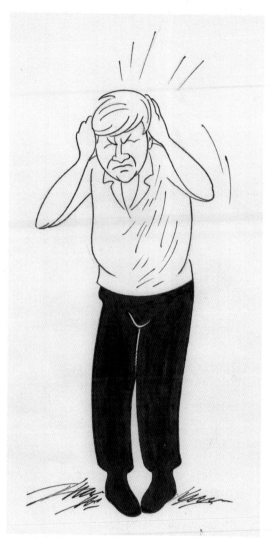

FIGURE 1.8 About half of irritable bowel syndrome patients suffer from periods of headache, which are believed to be caused by tension in the head and shoulder muscles

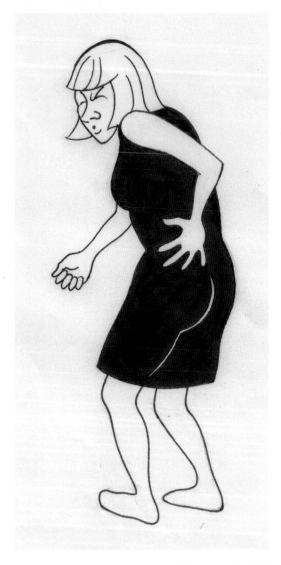

FIGURE 1.9 Diffuse muscle-related pain with sore points (fibromyalgia) can be associated with irritable bowel syndrome in some patients

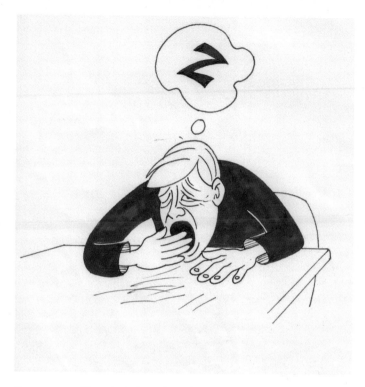

FIGURE 1.10 Chronic fatigue (i.e., fatigue that lasts for more than 6 months without any known medical reason) is also found in association with irritable bowel syndrome

Pain from the Urinary and Reproductive Organs

Reportedly 21–31 % of IBS patients have painful urination without any apparent cause. A small proportion of IBS patients also suffer from vaginal pain after sexual intercourse.

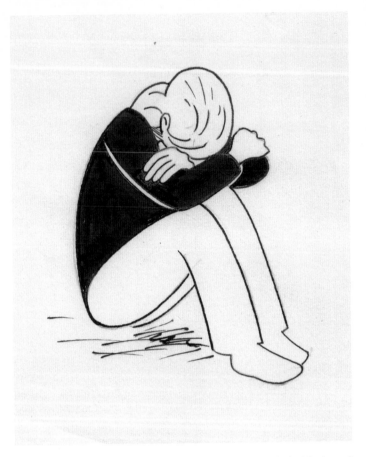

FIGURE 1.11 There exists an association between irritable bowel syndrome and depression, and some patients can suffer from periods of deep depression

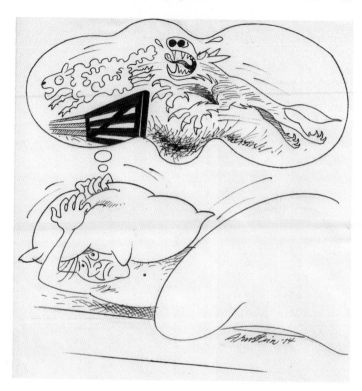

FIGURE 1.12 Some patients with irritable bowel syndrome suffer from sleeping difficulties

Chapter 2
The Digestive Tract and How It Works

Summary

- The digestive tract is an important organ, whose function is to break down the food we eat into small nutrients that are absorbed and distributed to the other organs of the body.
- The digestive tract consists of several segments: the mouth, esophagus, stomach, and the small and large bowels.
- All of the bowel functions are controlled and regulated by a local system of endocrine cells and nerve cells that lie within its walls [i.e., the neuroendocrine system (NES)].
- The NES operates independently from the central nervous system (the brain and spinal cord), but communicates and integrates with the brain and other parts of the nervous system.
- The first component of the NES is the endocrine cells, which are scattered among the cells lining the bowel lumen. These cells react to the contents of the bowel lumen, and especially nutrients, by releasing their hormones into the bloodstream.
- The bowel endocrine cells are abnormal in patients with IBS.

In order to understand the mechanisms underlying irritable bowel syndrome (IBS), it is necessary to have a basic knowledge of the digestive tract and its functions. The

M. El-Salhy et al., *Understanding and Controlling the Irritable Bowel*, DOI 10.1007/978-3-319-15642-2_2,
© Springer International Publishing Switzerland 2015

digestive tract is an important organ for the entire body. Its function is to break down the food we eat into small units of carbohydrates (monosaccharides), proteins (amino acids), fat (fatty acids), vitamins, and minerals, and to absorb these small units into the bloodstream, in which they are distributed to different organs of the body. The supply of these small units of carbohydrates, proteins, fat, vitamins, and minerals to the different organs of the body is necessary for those organs to function correctly. In other words, a well-functioning digestive tract is necessary for the wellbeing of the entire body.

The Gastrointestinal Tract and How It Functions

The gastrointestinal tract (Fig. 2.1) starts at the mouth, from which a long tube called the esophagus emerges. The esophagus leads to the stomach, which opens to the small bowel, which in turn continues to the large bowel. A common channel (duct) from the gallbladder and pancreas opens into the small bowel, delivering bile acid and pancreatic juice. The esophagus is about 20 cm long, the stomach is 30 cm long, the small bowel is about 6 m long, and the large bowel is about 1 m long, resulting in the gastrointestinal tract, being about 7.5 m long.

Biting, chewing, and moistening of the food with saliva take place in the mouth. The saliva contains chemical substances (enzymes) that start breaking down large molecules of carbohydrates to small units. The food is then transported along the esophagus to the stomach, where it typically remains for 4–6 h, during which time the food is mixed with the gastric juice, which contains enzymes that break down carbohydrates, proteins, and fats. The partially digested food then enters the first part of the small bowel, where it is mixed with bile acid and pancreatic juice, which contains several enzymes that complete the breakdown of carbohydrates, proteins, and fats. The small units of carbohydrates (monosaccharides), proteins (amino acids), and fats (fatty acids), as well as vitamins and minerals are absorbed into the blood as they pass through the rest of the small bowel.

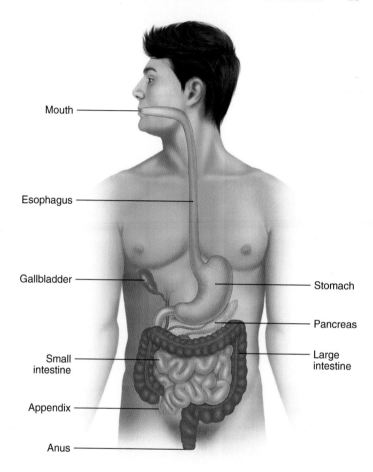

Mouth

Esophagus

Gallbladder

Stomach

Pancreas

Small
intestine

Large
intestine

Appendix

Anus

FIGURE 2.1 The digestive system starts at the mouth, which leads to
a long tube, the esophagus. The esophagus enters a sack, the stomach, which in turn opens into a long coiled tube, the small intestine.
Bile acids and pancreatic juice are emptied through a common duct
into the start of the small intestine. The small intestine leads to a
larger and shorter tube, the large intestine, which ends at the anus

The remains of the food enter the large bowel, where they are
concentrated by the removal of water and minerals. Finally, the
waste is expelled through the rectum as feces (Fig. 2.2).

The food at different stages of digestion and absorption is propelled along the esophagus and bowel via a movement called peristalsis (Fig. 2.3), which is brought about by rhythmic and coordinated contraction of the muscles in the walls of the gastrointestinal tract (beginning at the esophagus) behind the food and relaxation of those in front. The ability

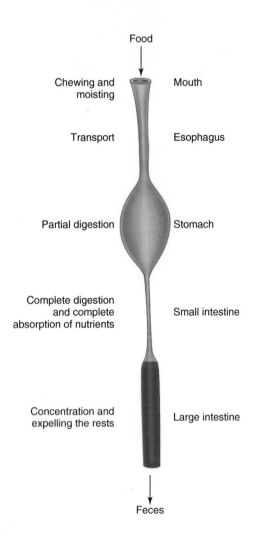

Food

Chewing and moisting — Mouth

Transport — Esophagus

Partial digestion — Stomach

Complete digestion and complete absorption of nutrients — Small intestine

Concentration and expelling the rests — Large intestine

Feces

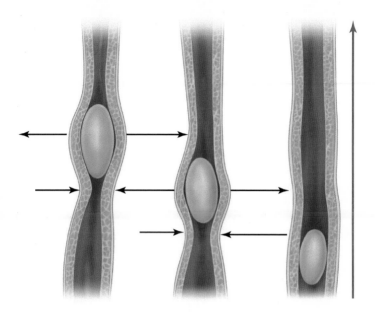

FIGURE 2.3 The gastrointestinal tract propels the digesting food from the mouth to the anus via a movement called peristalsis, which is a rhythmic and coordinated contraction of the muscles in the walls of the gastrointestinal tract behind the food and relaxation of those in front

FIGURE 2.2 The digestion of the food we eat and absorption of the nutrients in that food starts upon the food entering the mouth, where it is chewed and moistened with saliva, and then transported to the stomach through the esophagus. In the stomach, the food is mixed with the gastric juice, which partially digests it. The partially digested food then enters the small intestine, where it is mixed with the bile acids and pancreatic juice, which complete the digestion process. The digested nutrients pass through and are absorbed by the long small intestine. The remaining indigestible part of the food enters the large intestine, where it is concentrated by the removal of water and minerals. Finally, the waste is expelled through the anus as feces

of the gastrointestinal tract to propel the digesting food from the mouth to the anus is often referred to as motility.

Control and Regulation of Bowel Functions

All of the bowel functions are controlled and regulated by a local regulatory system within the bowel called the neuroendocrine system (NES). This regulatory system operates independently from the peripheral and central (brain and spinal cord) nervous systems, but it communicates and coordinates with the brain and the rest of the nervous system. The NES comprises two parts (Fig. 2.4) that interact and integrate with each other: endocrine cells (which secrete hormones into the bloodstream) and nerve cells (which secret neurotransmitter and neuromodulators). The endocrine cells are scattered among the cells lining the lumen of all parts of the gastrointestinal tract except for the esophagus (i.e., stomach and bowel; Figs. 2.5 and 2.6). These cells, which secrete about 15 different hormones and represent the largest endocrine gland of the body, send out tentacles to the gastrointestinal lumen that register the events in the lumen of the stomach and bowel, and respond to its contents, especially nutrients, by releasing specific hormones. We shall give two examples to illustrate this. First, if we eat fat, endocrine cells located in the upper part of the small bowel that secrete a hormone called cholecystokinin would sense the fat content in the small-bowel lumen, and in response release this hormone into the bloodstream. The cholecystokinin causes the gallbladder to empty gall salts into the small-bowel lumen, which will help to digest the fats. In a second example, if we eat proteins, another endocrine cell type located in the neighborhood of the cholecystokinin cells would sense the presence of proteins in the small-bowel cavity and release a hormone called secretin. Upon reaching the pancreas, secretin stimulates emptying of the pancreatic juice into the small bowel. Pancreatic juice contains enzymes that help to digest proteins.

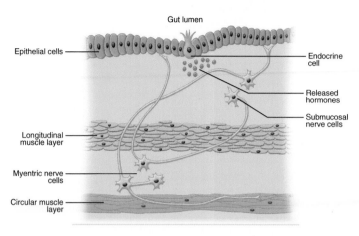

Gut lumen

Epithelial cells

Endocrine cell

Released hormones

Submucosal nerve cells

Longitudinal muscle layer

Myentric nerve cells

Circular muscle layer

FIGURE 2.4 The control and regulation of all of the bowel functions are achieved by a local regulatory system within the bowel called the neuroendocrine system (NES). This regulatory system operates independently from but communicates with the other parts of the nervous system. The NES comprises two types of cell that interact and integrate with each other: endocrine and nerve cells. The endocrine cells are scattered among the cells lining the lumen. The other part of the NES comprises nerve cells that are embedded in the gastrointestinal wall (the enteric nervous system) at two locations: (1) close to the gastrointestinal lumen (the submucosal plexus) and (2) within the muscle layers (the myenteric plexus)

The other part of the NES is nerve cells that are embedded in the gastrointestinal wall (the enteric nervous system) at two locations: (1) close to the gastrointestinal lumen (the submucosal plexus) and (2) within the muscle layers of the esophagus, stomach, and bowel (the myenteric plexus). These nerve cells interact and integrate with each other and with the gastrointestinal hormones secreted by the endocrine cells. Furthermore, they communicate with the brain (central nervous system) and with the autonomic nervous system (sympathetic and parasympathetic) divisions of both the central and peripheral nervous systems, which is responsible for the control of involuntary body functions such as the heartbeat, breathing, and digestion.

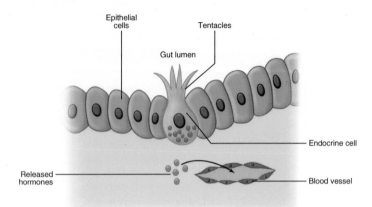

FIGURE 2.5 The endocrine cells are scattered among the cells lining the lumen of all parts of the gastrointestinal tract except for the esophagus. These cells secrete about 15 different hormones. They send out tentacles to the gastrointestinal lumen that register the events in the lumen of the stomach and bowel, and respond to its contents, especially nutrients, by releasing specific hormones. The released hormones reach the bloodstream through the underlying blood vessels, and also have a local effect on the neighboring endocrine cells and epithelial cells as well as the nerve cells of the enteric nervous system

Abnormal Functions of the Gastrointestinal Tract in Patients with IBS

Three abnormalities of gastrointestinal functions have been described in IBS patients: abnormal gastrointestinal motility, gastrointestinal hypersensitivity (visceral hypersensitivity), and abnormal gastrointestinal secretions. The gastrointestinal tract moves either slower or faster in patients with IBS than in healthy individuals. This abnormal motility has been found in all segments of the gastrointestinal tract other than the mouth, namely the esophagus, the stomach, and the small and large bowels. The visceral hypersensitivity experienced by IBS patients means that their bowel is more sensitive to stimuli such as pressure in the bowel lumen than in healthy

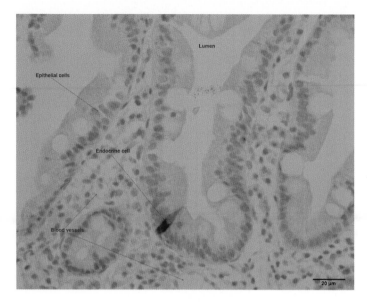

FIGURE 2.6 Gastrointestinal endocrine cells as seen under a light microscope (compare with Figure 2.5)

individuals. This can be exemplified by inserting a balloon into the anus or the large bowel and measuring the limits of pressure required to cause pain. These limits (threshold) are much lower in IBS patients than in healthy individuals. Moreover, it has been reported that the secretion of water and electrolytes (mostly sodium and potassium) into the gastrointestinal tract is abnormal in IBS patients.

Abnormalities in Bowel Endocrine Cells

Abnormalities in several of the endocrine cell types have been reported in the stomach and the small and large bowels of patients with IBS. These abnormalities appear to explain the aforementioned abnormalities in gastrointestinal functions that are found in IBS patients (i.e., abnormal gastrointestinal motility, gastrointestinal hypersensitivity, and abnormal gastrointestinal secretions).

Chapter 3
The Cause of Irritable Bowel Syndrome

Summary

- There is no convincing evidence that psychological factors affect the onset and/or progression of irritable bowel syndrome (IBS), but psychological factors such as stress can worsen the symptoms.
- The cause of IBS is not completely understood, but several factors seem to be involved in its development: heritability, environment and social learning, diet, large-bowel bacteria, low-grade inflammation, and abnormal bowel endocrine cells.
- We have postulated that IBS is caused by abnormalities in the gastrointestinal endocrine cells. These abnormalities are caused in turn by heritability, diet, composition of large-bowel bacteria, and low-grade inflammation.

In the absence of detectable somatic (i.e., physical) abnormalities in irritable bowel syndrome (IBS), it has been considered for a long time to be a psychological disorder caused by anxiety, depression, somatization (physical symptoms caused by psychological stress), or hypochondria. Although recent research has shown that there is no convincing evidence to support an effect of psychological factors on the onset and/or progression of IBS, stress can worsen the symptoms. Although the cause of IBS is not completely understood, several factors appear to be involved in its development,

M. El-Salhy et al., *Understanding and Controlling the Irritable Bowel*, DOI 10.1007/978-3-319-15642-2_3,
© Springer International Publishing Switzerland 2015

including heritability, environment and social learning, diet, composition of large-bowel bacteria, low-grade inflammation, and abnormal gastrointestinal endocrine cells.

Heritability

About one-third of IBS patients have a family history of the disorder. Several studies have shown that IBS is common among the relatives of IBS patients. Studies on twins have shown that the chances of one twin having IBS if the other twin has IBS are greater if they are identical twins (i.e., formed from a single egg) than if they are fraternal twins (i.e., formed from two eggs). Moreover, genetic studies have provided evidence for a hereditary component in IBS.

Environment and Social Learning

There is some evidence that the illness behavior (i.e., the manner in which an individual monitor the structure and functions of his body, interpret symptoms, take an action, and make use of healthcare facilities) in a family contributes to the causes of IBS. Having a mother with IBS accounts for as much as genetic factors. Of course this raises the question as to whether IBS is caused (1) by the possession of half a set of genes from a mother with IBS or (2) by social learning.

Diet

Most patients with IBS find that certain foodstuffs trigger their symptoms, and often make a conscious decision to avoid these foodstuffs, which include milk and dairy products, wheat products, onion, garlic, peas, beans, hot spices, cabbage, smoked products, fried food, and caffeine. The effect of these foods on IBS symptoms is not due to an allergy or intolerance, but other factors as explained below.

Some foodstuffs are rich in short-chain carbohydrates, the so-called fermentable oligosaccharides, disaccharides, monosaccharides, and polyols (FODMAPs; Table 3.1). These carbohydrates are poorly absorbed, and a significant portion enters the distal part of the small bowel and the large bowel. On entering the large bowel, they increase the osmotic pressure and become a substrate for bacterial fermentation, which results in gas production, distention of the abdomen, and abdominal discomfort or pain.

For a long time it has been believed that IBS is caused by low intake of dietary fiber, and hence a standard recommendation for patients has been to increase the dietary fiber intake. However, recent research has shown that there are two types of dietary fiber: water-soluble and not water-soluble (Table 3.2). When soluble fiber dissolves in water it forms a gel, while insoluble fiber passes intact through the gastrointestinal tract, reaching the distal part of the small bowel and large bowel where, as for FODMAPs, it increases the osmotic pressure and becomes a substrate for bacterial fermentation, with the same results as for FODMAPs. Therefore, rather than improving IBS symptoms, increasing the intake of nonsoluble fiber will increase abdominal pain, bloating, and distension. Conversely, increasing the intake of soluble fiber will improve the overall IBS symptoms. In addition to its beneficial effects on IBS symptoms, soluble fiber aids in achieving healthy weight by delaying stomach emptying and reducing appetite, probably through the appetite hormone ghrelin. It also has a beneficial effect on insulin sensitivity in type 2 diabetes and lowers the level of blood cholesterol, thus protecting against cardiovascular diseases. While unfortunately there are no foods that contain only soluble or insoluble fiber, their relative proportions do vary between foodstuffs.

Large-Bowel Bacteria

Most bacteria in the bowel are localized to the large bowel, which is colonized with between 300 and 500 different bacteria. Each individual has his/her own unique specific

TABLE 3.1 The most common foodstuffs with a high content of fermentable oligosaccharides, disaccharides, monosaccharides, and polyols (FODMAPs)

Oligosaccharides: fructans and galactans	Disaccharides: lactose	Monosaccharides: fructose	Polyols
Wheat and rye: *bread, pasta, couscous, crackers, biscuits*	*Milk and dairy products*: *cheeses, yoghurt*	Honey and sweeteners containing fructose such as corn syrup	
Sweeteners: inulin			Sweeteners: <u>sorbitol, mannitol, xylitol, isomalt, maltitol, and other sweeteners with names ending in "-ol"</u>
Vegetables: *onions, garlic, leeks, spring onion, paprika,* <u>beans</u>, lentils, <u>red kidney beans</u>, Brussels sprout, <u>broccoli</u>, *cabbage*, asparagus, beetroot, artichokes, fennel, okra, peas, shallots			Vegetables: *mushrooms*, snow peas, cauliflower, avocado

Fruits: watermelon, peaches, apples, persimmon, custard	Fruits: apples, pears, peaches, mangos, watermelon, sugar-snap peas, dried fruits, fruit juice, tinned fruit in natural juice	Fruits: watermelon, apples, nashi pears, apricots, longan, cherries, lychees, nectarines, peaches, prunes

Note: Irritable bowel syndrome (IBS) patients usually avoid the foodstuffs in *italics*, while they tend to overconsume those that are underlined

TABLE 3.2 Example foodstuffs that contain predominantly soluble or insoluble fiber

Soluble dietary fiber	Insoluble dietary fiber
Oatmeal, oat cereal, psyllium	Whole wheat, whole grains, wheat bran, corn bran, seeds, nuts, barley, couscous, brown rice
Vegetables: beans, dried peas, lentils, flaxseeds, nuts, carrots, cucumbers, celery, soybeans	Vegetables: bulgur, zucchini, broccoli, cabbage, onions, tomatoes, green beans, dark leafy vegetables, root vegetable skins
Fruits: apples, oranges, pears, strawberries, blueberries	Fruits: raisins, grapes

composition of these bacteria. The factors that determine the number and kinds of bacteria in each individual are genetic disposition (certain bacteria prefer certain individuals), the diet, climate change i.e., moving from a hot climate to cold climate and vice versa, stress level, age, disease presence, and use of medications (especially antibiotics).

The bacteria that populate the large bowel can be grossly divided into "bad" and "good" bacteria. The bad bacteria damage the membrane lining the cavity of the bowel either directly or indirectly via the production of toxins (poisons); examples of such bacteria are *Campylobacter*, *Salmonella*, *Shigella* species, and *Vibrio comma*. These bacteria can cause various diseases with symptoms such as diarrhea (including bloody diarrhea), bowel cramps, and fever. In IBS, the major bad bacteria are *Clostridium* species, which break down undigested sugars and fiber entering the large bowel and produce gas, resulting in abdominal destination and pain or discomfort. The good bacteria, such as *Lactobacilli* and *Bifidobacterium* species, benefit their host in several ways:

1. They produce several vitamins, such as B_1, B_6, B_9, and K, that can be absorbed and used by the body.
2. They produce enzymes that help us to absorb certain electrolytes such as calcium, magnesium, and iron.

3. They create a barrier (wall) around mucous membranes, thus protecting them.
4. They break down the waste in the large bowel to short-chain fatty acids, which are the main energy source for the membrane lining the bowel lumen.
5. They break down nonabsorbed sugars and nonabsorbed fiber without producing gas.
6. Some of these bacteria produce substances that kill the bad bacteria and neutralize their toxins.
7. Some of these bacteria produce substances that protect against inflammation and enhance the immune defense in ways we don't yet understand.

The large-bowel bacteria differ between IBS patients and healthy individuals. *Lactobacilli* and *Bifidobacterium* species are less populous in patients with IBS than in healthy individuals, while *Clostridium* species are more abundant in IBS patients. Furthermore, oral intake of the beneficial *Lactobacilli* and *Bifidobacterium* species does not result in permanent colonization of the large bowel; rather, they disappear from the large bowel after only 1 week.

Low-Grade Inflammation

Some patients, and especially those with postinfectious IBS (see Chap. 4), have a low-grade inflammation in the wall of the large bowel that is manifested by an increase in the number of immune cells in the area close to the bowel lumen. There is a general consensus that this inflammation plays a role in the development of IBS, at least in a subgroup of patients.

Abnormal Bowel Endocrine Cells

Recent studies have shown that several types of endocrine cells in the gastrointestinal tract are abnormal. These abnormalities have been found in the endocrine cells in different segments of the gastrointestinal tract, namely the stomach and the small and large bowels. As mentioned previously (Chap. 2), the gastrointestinal endocrine cells are the first line in the local regulatory system, the neuroendocrine system (NES), which controls all gastrointestinal functions. These cells initiate a series of events in response to those occurring in the gastrointestinal lumen. Interestingly, the abnormalities in these endocrine cell types can explain other gastrointestinal function abnormalities observed in IBS patients, namely gastrointestinal hypersensitivity, abnormal gastrointestinal motility, and abnormal gastrointestinal secretion (see Chap. 2). We believe that the abnormalities in the gastrointestinal endocrine cell in IBS play a central role in the development of IBS.

Hypothesis

We have proposed the following hypothesis to explain the cause of IBS (Fig. 3.1) that considers all of the factors known to play a role in IBS: IBS is caused by disturbance in the endocrine cells of the gastrointestinal tract that are brought about by hereditary factors, the composition of large-bowel bacteria, dietary factors, and low-grade inflammation within the large bowel. The following recent data support this hypothesis:

1. Genetic factors influence the gastrointestinal endocrine system, probably through the development of different endocrine cells from the multipotent stem cells.
2. The change in large-bowel bacterial composition alters the gastrointestinal endocrine cells.
3. The change in diet in IBS patients changes the density of endocrine cells.
4. Inflammation in the large bowel with subsequent invasion of immune cells alters the density and activities of the large-bowel endocrine cells.

Stress and IBS

There are different types of stress: physical (e.g., fatigue, serious infection), or psychological (e.g., relationship conflicts or

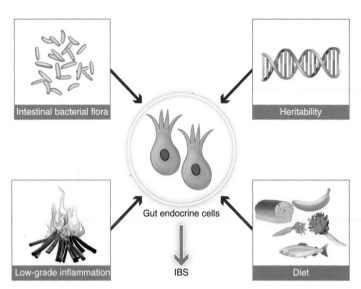

FIGURE 3.1 Heritability, diet, low-grade inflammation, and intestinal bacterial flora are factors that are known to be involved in the development of irritable bowel syndrome. We have proposed a hypothesis that IBS is caused by a disturbance in the endocrine cells of the gastrointestinal tract that is brought about by hereditary factors, dietary factors, the composition of large-bowel bacteria, and low-grade inflammation within the large bowel

stressful life events). Stress does not cause IBS, but it does worsen the symptoms. We believe that this worsening of symptoms is caused by an interaction between stress hormones such as cortisone and adrenalin, and gastrointestinal hormones. In support of our assumption, physical activities that increase the release of endorphins and encephalin—the so-called "happiness" hormones—have been found to relieve IBS symptoms. Moreover, IBS symptoms appear to be exacerbated in women during menstruation and diminished during pregnancy, indicating another interaction between the sex hormones and the gastrointestinal hormones.

Chapter 4
How is Irritable Bowel Syndrome Diagnosed?

Summary

- There is no blood test or examination for the definitive diagnosis of irritable bowel (IBS). Instead, diagnosis is based on the exclusion of gastrointestinal diseases that can produce symptoms similar to those of IBS.
- In order to avoid performing extensive expensive and troublesome tests and examinations, a symptom-based diagnosis has been introduced: the Rome criteria.
- The Rome criteria were introduced more than 20 years ago, but they are still not commonly used in everyday clinical practice.
- In our clinical practice we perform gastroscopy and colonoscopy in all IBS patients to exclude the gastrointestinal diseases that can mimic IBS due to their similar symptoms.
- We propose using the abnormalities observed in the gastrointestinal endocrine cells for the diagnosis of IBS.

Since there are no blood tests or other examinations that are diagnostic for irritable bowel syndrome (IBS), this condition is generally diagnosed by exclusion. This means that gastrointestinal diseases that can also give rise to the symptoms exhibited in IBS are excluded by performing several tests and examinations that are diagnostic of those diseases.

M. El-Salhy et al., *Understanding and Controlling the Irritable Bowel*, DOI 10.1007/978-3-319-15642-2_4,
© Springer International Publishing Switzerland 2015

Symptom-Based Diagnosis

The exclusion approach to reach the IBS diagnosis is expensive and subjects the patients to troublesome, racking, and often painful examinations. Therefore, several attempts have been made to achieve a positive diagnosis based on clinical symptoms similar to those used in psychiatric and rheumatic diseases. In 1988, these attempts culminated in the introduction of the Rome I criteria by an international panel of experts. These criteria were followed by refinements in 1999 (Rome II criteria) and in 2006 (Rome III criteria).

The criteria for the diagnosis of IBS as described by Rome III are intermittent abdominal pain/discomfort on at least 3 days per month in the last 3 months together with two of the following three criteria: improvement on defecation, change in stool frequency, or change in the stool form. To exclude other organic diseases with similar symptoms, patients should not express any additional potentially alarming symptoms such as rectal bleeding, anemia, loss of body weight, fever, or signs of inflammation. IBS patients are divided according to Rome III criteria into three subtypes on the basis of differences in the predominant bowel habits: diarrhea-predominant, constipation-predominant, or a mixture of both diarrhea and constipation. The main goal of this subdivision was to facilitate treatment of the symptoms. However, this subdivision is unstable and interchangeable, with more than 75 % of IBS patients switching from one subtype to another over time.

Even though more than 2 decades have passed since the introduction of symptom-based IBS diagnosis according Rome criteria, it is still not used in everyday practice. The difficulties in applying these criteria in real clinical practice are attributable to both patients and physicians. Patients with IBS who seek healthcare often expect to be investigated thoroughly as they are worried that their symptoms are being caused by a serious disease. It is therefore not sufficient to dismiss these patients without further investigation. Experience has shown that these patients repetitively seek healthcare providers until they feel that their concerns have been taken seriously and they have been investigated thoroughly. As for the physicians, they are concerned about missing serious organic diseases and are not comfortable reaching a diagnosis based on symptoms that can also be manifested by other gastrointestinal diseases.

The gastrointestinal conditions that mimic IBS are celiac disease, microscopic colitis (inflammation that can only be detected by microscopic examination of tissue samples from the large bowel), inflammatory bowel diseases, large-bowel cancer, bile-acid malabsorption, bacterial overgrowth, and pelvic-floor disorders. The rates of celiac disease, microscopic colitis, inflammatory bowel diseases, and large-bowel cancer in IBS patients diagnosed according to symptom-based criteria reportedly lie in the ranges 0.04–4.7 %, 0.7–1.5 %, 0.4–1.9 %, and 0.02–0.5 %, respectively. Moreover, bile-acid malabsorption affects 30–50 % of patients with chronic diarrhea. Thus, a considerable number of patients diagnosed with IBS using symptom-based criteria could suffer from other organic diseases that require treatments other than that for IBS. These patients would be misdiagnosed if further investigations were not performed. Regardless of the paucity of these patients relative to the IBS population, they should not be misdiagnosed and denied the proper treatment.

In our clinical practice, we perform only a few examinations in addition to the symptom-based Rome III criteria. All IBS patients undergo a complete physical examination and are investigated by way of blood tests to exclude inflammatory, liver, endocrine, or any other systemic diseases. Furthermore, we perform a gastroscopy (see Appendix A), during which we take tissue samples of the small bowel to exclude celiac disease, and colonoscopy (see Appendix B) during which we take tissue samples from different parts of the large bowel to exclude inflammatory bowel diseases, microscopic colitis, and large-bowel cancer. In a few patients we perform other examinations to exclude bile-acid malabsorption, bacterial overgrowth, and pelvic floor disorders.

The IBS Types

There are three types of IBS: sporadic (nonspecific), postinfectious IBS, and inflammatory-bowel-diseases-associated IBS. Patients with sporadic IBS are those who have had symptoms for a long time and are without any associated events, in particular gastrointestinal or other infections. Postinfectious IBS occurs after a sudden onset of IBS symptoms following a bout of gastroenteritis in individuals who have previously had no gastrointestinal complaints. Inflammatory-bowel-disease-associated IBS is diagnosed in patients with inflammatory bowel diseases who display IBS symptoms during bowel-inflammation-free periods. Postinfectious IBS reportedly accounts for 6–17 % of all IBS patients, and inflammatory-bowel-disease-associated IBS occurs in about 50 % of all patients with inflammatory bowel diseases.

Tests and Examinations for the Diagnosis of IBS

Several attempts have been made to find a test or examination that will provide a positive diagnosis of IBS. Tests for detecting the abnormalities that occur in IBS patients, such as gastrointestinal dysmotility, gastrointestinal hypersensitivity, autonomic nervous reactivity, and inflammation, have been considered, but thus far none has been found to be useful for IBS diagnosis.

We have proposed that the small bowel cell density of chromogranin A, which is a common marker for endocrine cells, could be used as a test for the diagnosis of IBS—for which it has been found to be reliable. Moreover, this test is an inexpensive, simple, and easy-to-use method that does not require sophisticated equipment or considerable experience, which means it can be performed in small pathology laboratories. In addition, the cell densities of two other cells in the large bowel that contain the hormones peptide YY and somatostatin have proven to be a good test for the diagnosis of IBS. These tests are also easy to perform and inexpensive.

As mentioned above, in our practice we take tissue samples from the duodenum during the gastroscopy procedure to exclude celiac disease; these same tissue samples can be used for the chromogranin A test. Similarly, the tissue samples obtained from the large bowel during colonoscopy can be used for the analysis of peptide YY and somatostatin cells. Thus, applying these proposed histological tests does not require the patient to undergo additional examinations.

Chapter 5
Treatment Options Without Medication

Summary

- Nonmedication therapies are used equally by general practitioners and specialists, but patients with irritable bowel syndrome (IBS) have greater confidence in these treatments than in medications. Nonmedication therapies is also proven to be more effective than medication treatments.

- Nonmedication therapies include the delivery of IBS-oriented information, dietary management, regular exercise, probiotic intake, hypnotherapy, acupuncture, relaxation training, cognitive behavioral therapy, and psychodynamic and psychological therapies.

- The delivery of IBS-oriented information, dietary management, regular exercise, probiotic intake, and hypnotherapy exert documented effects on IBS symptoms and patient quality of life.

- The combination of delivery of IBS-oriented information, dietary management, probiotic intake, and regular exercise has an additive effect, reducing IBS symptoms and improving the quality of life in patients with mild and moderate IBS.

- Gastrointestinal-directed hypnotherapy is the approach of choice for those with severe IBS.

M. El-Salhy et al., *Understanding and Controlling the Irritable Bowel*, DOI 10.1007/978-3-319-15642-2_5,
© Springer International Publishing Switzerland 2015

Irritable bowel syndrome (IBS) can be treated with or without involving medication (see Chap. 6). General practitioners and specialists use both approaches to the same degree, but patients with IBS have greater confidence in the nonmedication therapies than in the medications. It has also been found that the nonmedication approach is more effective than that involving medications. The nonmedication therapies include one or more of the following: delivery of IBS-oriented information, dietary management, regular exercise, probiotic intake, gastrointestinal-directed hypnotherapy, acupuncture, herbal therapy, cognitive behavioral therapy, psychodynamic interpersonal therapy, relaxation training, and psychological treatment.

IBS-Oriented Information

Studies conducted on IBS patients to establish how much they know about IBS have revealed that about 50 % believe that IBS is caused by a lack of digestive enzymes, and about 50 % believe that it is a form of colitis (inflammation in the large bowel). Moreover, many IBS patients believe that their condition will deteriorate with age, and that it can develop into colitis, malnutrition, or cancer.

Most IBS patients are interested in learning about which foods to avoid, the causes of IBS, coping strategies, and medications for IBS. They are also interested in finding out whether or not they will have to live with IBS for the rest of their life, and in reading research studies on the condition. Information and education are both requested by IBS patients and have proven to be beneficial. Thus, a thorough 15-min verbal explanation of the diagnosis and underlying mechanisms of IBS by a gastroenterologist during the first consultation was found to reduce self-perceptions of impairment in daily functioning. Furthermore, a structured 3-h IBS educational class for patients with IBS was reported to improve symptoms and some health-promoting behaviors. A 12-h structured IBS educational program, which included a

2-h informative session with a gastroenterologist, was found to improve both the IBS symptoms and quality of life of patients. Moreover, an effective physician–patient relationship that provides both reassurance and a thorough explanation of the IBS disorder has been found to reduce the use of healthcare resources and the fear of cancer. We believe that information provided by the healthcare provider is important to reassure the patient and to help them to cope with their condition.

Dietary Management

Diet plays an important role in the development of IBS symptoms (see Chap. 3). Several studies have shown that restricting FODMAPs intake reduces the symptoms of IBS (Fig. 5.1). However, it is rather difficult to completely avoid FODMAPs over long periods. In our experience, IBS patients' tolerance to FODMAPs differs considerably from individual to individual, probably because of differences in the composition of large-bowel bacteria. In our clinic, some IBS patients can tolerate small amounts of garlic and onions, while others cannot tolerate these items in any amounts; this also applies to bread, milk, and dairy products. The IBS patient should test the different items listed in Table 3.1 and elucidate how much she/he tolerate. Furthermore, there are many alternatives to FODMAPs-containing foodstuffs that can be consumed by IBS patients (Table 5.1), and by doing so it is possible for IBS patients to lead a normal everyday life (Figs. 5.2, 5.3, 5.4, 5.5, 5.6 and 5.7).

There are two other important dietary factors that affect IBS symptoms. As mentioned in Chap. 3, the nutrient content of the gastrointestinal tract causes the release of different gastrointestinal hormones that regulate gastrointestinal motility, the secretion of different enzymes, and the sensibility of the gastrointestinal tract. The relative proportions of carbohydrates, protein, and fats that we ingest affect the secretion of these gastrointestinal hormones. Furthermore,

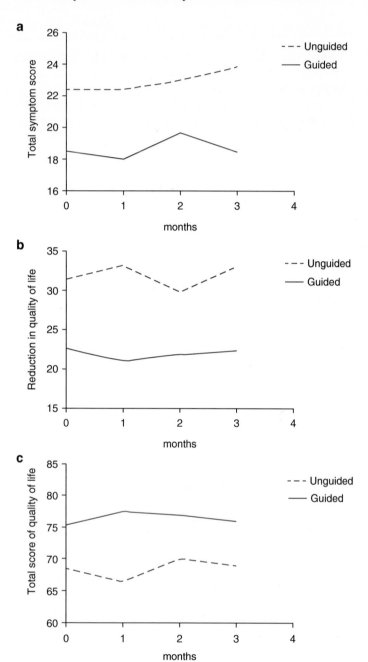

what we eat represents the substrate for the growth of different large-bowel bacteria, so that the types of food that we eat (prebiotics) favor the growth of certain types of bacteria over others.

The consumption of dietary fiber accelerates the passage of bowel contents and increases the pressure in the large bowel, therefore playing a role in the management of IBS symptoms, and particularly constipation. However, it is necessary to distinguish between water-insoluble and water-soluble fiber, given that soluble fiber improves symptoms whereas insoluble fiber worsens them. IBS patients should therefore be recommended to increase their intake of foods rich in soluble fiber (Table 3.2). In the clinic, as for FODMAPs, the tolerance to insoluble fiber varies widely between IBS patients, also possibly due to differences in the composition of intestinal bacteria between patients. Furthermore, consuming foods supplemented with probiotics increases a patient's tolerance to FODMAPs and insoluble fiber.

Regular Exercise

Regular exercise reduces IBS symptoms and improves the patient's quality of life. Based on clinical experience, physicians often recommend regular exercise for IBS patients. The effects of physical activity on IBS patients were attributed to promoting overall wellbeing. However, physical activity has

FIGURE 5.1 The total symptom score according to the Birmingham irritable bowel syndrome Symptom Score questionnaire (**a**), reduction in the quality of life according to the Short-Form Nepean Dyspepsia Index questionnaire (**b**), and quality of life according to the Irritable Bowel Syndrome Quality of Life questionnaire (**c**) in 36 IBS patients without any restrictions in the intake of fermentable oligosaccharides, disaccharides, monosaccharides, and polyols (FODMAPs; unguided), and in 48 IBS patients, who received dietary guidance with restriction of FODMAPs intake (guided). All 84 patients were followed-up over a period of 3 months. Unpublished data

TABLE 5.1 Alternative foodstuffs with low contents of FODMAPs

Oligosaccharides: fructans and galactans	Disaccharides: lactose	Monosaccharides: fructose	Polyols
Spelt and spelt-based products, rice, corn	Lactose-free milk and dairy products, rice milk, hard cheeses	Sweeteners, maple syrup, golden syrup	Sweeteners: sugar, glucose, other sweeteners with names not ending in "-ol"
		Fruits: bananas, blueberries, oranges, mandarins, kiwifruit, grapes, grapefruit, honeydew melon, durian, passion fruit, raspberries, strawberries	Fruits: bananas, blueberries, mandarins, oranges, kiwifruit, grapes, grapefruit, honey-dew melon, durian, passion fruit, rasp-berries, strawberries
Vegetables: *garlic-infused oil*, carrot, celery, corn, eggplant, lettuce, bamboo shoots, bok choy, capsicum, green beans, chives, pumpkin, silver beet			

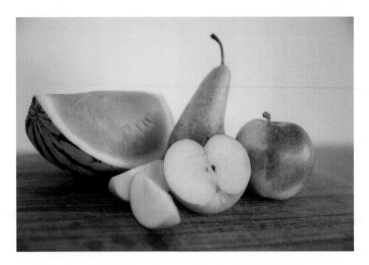

FIGURE 5.2 An illustration of some of the fruits that are rich in FODMAPs and/or insoluble fiber and should be avoided by irritable bowel syndrome patients

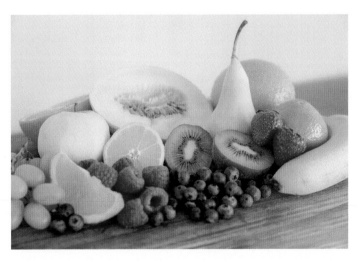

FIGURE 5.3 Although irritable bowel syndrome patients must avoid some fruits that are rich in FODMAPs, there are many delicious fruits that are poor in FODMAPs and hence that they can eat, as illustrated here

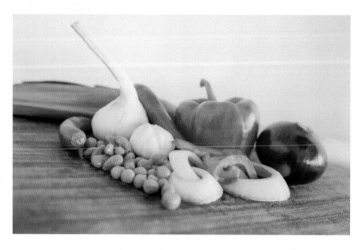

FIGURE 5.4 Some of the vegetables that are rich in FODMAPs and/ or insoluble fiber, and hence should be avoided by irritable bowel syndrome patients

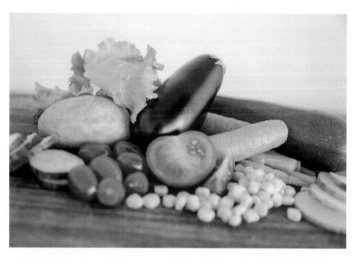

FIGURE 5.5 There are many vegetables that are poor in FODMAPS and/or insoluble fiber, and therefore can be consumed by irritable bowel syndrome patients, some of which are illustrated here

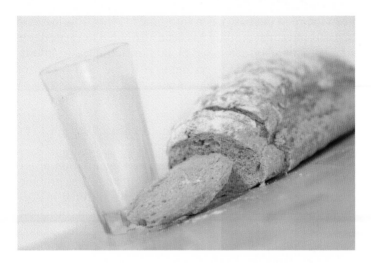

FIGURE 5.6 Bread (especially if it contains insoluble fiber) and milk are two of the food items that should be avoided by irritable bowel syndrome patients, since they are rich in FODMAPs

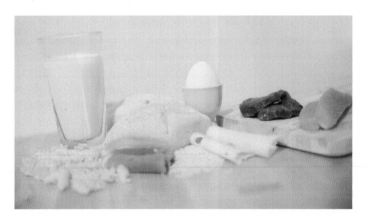

FIGURE 5.7 Lactose-free milk, spelt bread, and spelt pasta can be consumed by IBS patients. This picture also shows various other food items that can also be consumed by IBS patients

been found to increase gastrointestinal motility. This increase in gastrointestinal motility has been attributed to vagus nerve stimulation and/or decreased blood flow to the gastrointestinal tract, which leads to an increase in the distribution of important gastrointestinal hormones.

Probiotics and Prebiotics

According to the Food and Agriculture Organization of the United Nations and the World Health Organization, probiotics are live microorganisms that when administered in adequate amounts confer a health benefit upon the host. Probiotics include bacteria or yeasts from the genera *Lactobacillus*, *Bidifobacterium*, and *Saccharomyces*. The probiotics available on the market contain either single bacterial strains or a mixture of strains, and are available in the form of capsules, powders, yoghurts, and fermented milks. In order to exert their beneficial effects, they must be well tolerated for human consumption, and they must survive transit through the stomach and small bowel. The effects attributed to probiotics are enhancement of the host's anti-inflammatory and immune responses through stimulating the release of anti-inflammatory cytokines, improve the epithelial cell barrier, inhibit bacterial translocation and growth, inhibit the adhesion of viruses, and inactivate bile acids (see Chap. 3).

Treatment with a single probiotic preparation or with a probiotic mixture can improve IBS symptoms. The effect depends upon the preparation used, with some products appearing to be more effective than others. The bacteria *Bifidobacterium infantis* 35624, *Bifidobacterium Lactis DN-173-010*, *L. plantrum*, *L. GG*, *L. acidophilus*, and *S. faecium* have proven particularly effective. These bacteria reduce the number of sulfite-reducing *Clostridia* species, which are known to produce gas during the fermentation of nutrients; they consequently improve the IBS symptoms of flatulence, bloating, and abdominal distension. Furthermore, they have anti-inflammatory effects; modulation of the immune response might be an important factor in this regard. However, probiotics are not potent enough to be used alone, especially in patients with severe symptoms.

In clinical practice, IBS patients observe a relapse of the IBS symptoms as soon as they stop taking probiotics. This is in agreement with the finding that certain bacteria (e.g., *Lactobacillus acidophilus*) vanish from the feces 1 week after intake cessation. Thus, probiotics should be taken continuously.

Prebiotics are defined as nondigestible, fermentable food components that result in the selective stimulation and/or activity of one or a limited number of microbial genera/species in the gastrointestinal microbiota that confer health benefits upon the host. Prebiotics are only fermented by a limited number of genera/species, which subsequently increase in number driven by natural selection from the carbon and energy provided by prebiotics. The benefit and use of prebiotics in IBS are not yet clear, but represent a potential tool for the management of IBS.

Stord Hospital Combined Program

A program combining information, dietary management, probiotic intake, and regular exercise was implemented at Stord Hospital in 2005, and has so far been applied to more than 1,000 patients with IBS. This program comprises a 60-min consultation with a gastroenterologist, two 60-min sessions each with a nurse with special education in IBS, gastroscopy and colonoscopy with tissue biopsy sampling, and finally, a 30-min concluding consultation with the same gastroenterologist.

In the first consultation with a gastroenterologist, a complete physical examination and blood tests are conducted to exclude inflammation, infection, or other organic disease, and gastroscopy and colonoscopy are scheduled. The patients are informed verbally about IBS, as described in Table 5.2, including an explanation of the beneficial effects of combin-

TABLE 5.2 The information provided to irritable bowel syndrome (IBS) patients during the first consultation with a gastroenterologist through the Stord Hospital combined program

---

IBS is recognized as an illness and is a common disorder in the population.

It is more common in women than in men.

Although IBS can cause a considerable reduction in quality of life, it is not known to develop into a serious disease or to shorten life.

IBS is a chronic disorder.

The type and intensity of symptoms fluctuate; that is, there will be good and bad days.

The possible causes of IBS are explained.

The possible coexistence of other gastrointestinal and/or non-bowel-related symptoms in patients with IBS.

A thorough explanation of how a physical examination, blood tests, gastroscopy, and colonoscopy can exclude other diseases in these patients.

It is clearly stated that there is no miracle cure. A detailed account is given of the treatment options, and that a nonmedication approach could be sufficient and could be combined with medications on bad days.

Intensive research is ongoing worldwide, and our understanding of this disorder increases every day, and this will hopefully lead to new treatment possibilities.

---

ing dietary management, probiotic intake, and regular exercise; they are also provided with a pamphlet containing this information.

During the first session with the nurse, information regarding the role of diet in IBS and healthy eating habits healthy is given. The patients are instructed to avoid poorly absorbed FODMAPs and foodstuffs containing significant amounts of nonsoluble fiber, and are informed about the alternative foodstuffs that they should consumed (see Table 5.3). The provided table of alternatives was kept intentionally short so as to maximize its manageability. Furthermore, the patients are asked to try a carbohydrate-, protein-, or fat-rich/poor diet with the intention of reducing the amounts of bowel gas produced (since this causes abdominal pain/discomfort) and to reduce/increase the release of gastrointestinal hormones. This information is provided verbally and using charts and illustrative drawings. The patients are asked to keep a daily diary in which they record the time of eating/drinking, and the types of food and drinks that they ingest. Moreover, they report in the diary the occurrence of pain, abdominal distention, and the stool frequency and consistency. This is performed for at least 2 weeks prior to the second session. Pain and abdominal distention are graded as mild, moderate, or severe. In the second sessions the nurse goes through the diary with the patient, and together they design a suitable diet for the patient.

In the last consultation with the gastroenterologist, the information given under the program is summarized, and the patient is informed of the results of the gastroscopy and colonoscopy procedures and the blood tests. The physician answers the patient's questions, emphasizes that the symptoms will fluctuate over time, and provides the patient with a means of rescue during the bad days. On bad days, it is recommended that patients take dimetikon (200 mg) capsules to protect against abdominal bloating and distension, to exercise and/or to take medication against diarrhea or constipation. The patient is left to choose the type of exercise him/herself; for example, some patients choose to take long walks, while others use an indoor (stationary) bicycle. Patients report that exercise relieves abdominal pain and releases bowel gas.

The patients who have participated in this program have reported considerable improvements in their lifes: some were able to restore broken relationships, while others had returned to work after a long period of sick leave or had returned to the education program from which they had dropped out due

TABLE 5.3 General dietary advice to irritable bowel syndrome (IBS) patients according to Stord Hospital combined program

Food to avoid	Food allowed
Flour and flour-based products	Spelt and spelt-based products
Onions	Rice
Garlic	Potatoes
Paprika	Meat
Beans	Fish
Peas	Chicken
Avocado	Fat and oils
Artichokes	Carrots
Broccoli	Apples and pears (peeled)
Cabbage	Citrus fruits
Rutabaga	Bananas
Watermelon	Raspberries, blueberries, and strawberries
Carbonated beverages (soda)	Honeydew melon
Light products (food containing artificial sweeteners)	Kiwifruit and passion fruit
Alcohol: beer and whisky	Tomatoes
	Lettuce
	Lactose-free milk and dairy products
	Coffee and tea
	Chocolate
	Alcohol: corn beer and beverages
	Probiotic supplements

to their condition. We have followed up 143 patients for 2 years after they participated in this program, and recorded their symptoms and quality of life. These IBS patients experienced a reduction in symptoms and an improvement in the quality of life (Fig. 5.8), which were maintained throughout the follow-up period. These findings support the additive effect of combining several nonmedication approaches in a short health program.

Gastrointestinal-Directed Hypnotherapy

Gastrointestinal-directed hypnotherapy improves the symptoms, quality of life, and psychological status of IBS patients. These effects are sustained over time, for at least 5 years. However, these results were obtained in patients with mostly refractory IBS (patients with severe symptoms and a long duration of IBS) and were highly selected and motivated IBS patients. Hence, the results cannot be generalized to all IBS patients. The results of this treatment vary considerably between different centers, and should therefore be restricted to a few centers and reserved for severe forms of IBS.

This therapy uses hypnotic induction, progressive relaxation, and imagery directed toward the control and normalization of gastrointestinal functions. It also aims to teach the patients autohypnosis to enable them to manage their own condition. However, occasional refresher sessions are required. Gastrointestinal-directed hypnotherapy typically requires a total of 6–12 sessions, each between 30 and 60 min long, over a period of several months. It is demanding and requires the patient's cooperation, which may explain why the dropout rates are relatively high.

The effect of hypnotherapy appears to be attributable to activation of certain areas of the brain, and especially the anterior cingulate cortex, since hypnotic reduction of pain is associated with a reduction in the activation of this brain region.

FIGURE 5.8 The symptom score according to Birmingham irritable bowel syndrome Symptom Score questionnaire (**a**), reduction in the quality of life according to the 36-item Short Form questionnaire (**b**), and quality of life according to the the Irritable Bowel Syndrome Quality of Life questionnaire (**c**) in 143 patients who submitted to a health program comprising reassurance, diet management, probiotics intake, and regular exercise. These patients were followed up over a period of 2 years (Data from El-Salhy et al. *Gastroenterology Insights* 2010;2:21–26)

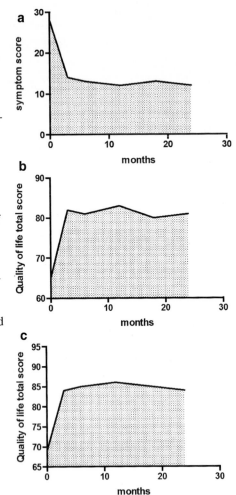

Acupuncture

Acupuncture is an ancient traditional Chinese medical practice. The theory behind acupuncture is the belief that energy or the life force "qi" runs through the body in channels, or "meridians." Qi is believed to be essential for health, and any disruption of its flow causes symptoms and disease. Disruption in the flow of qi can be corrected by acupuncture at certain identifiable locations called "acupoints." In modern times, the effect of acupuncture on pain is thought to be caused by its ability to release the body's own (endogenous) morphines: endorphins and encephalin. The effect on IBS seems to be caused by altering visceral (gastrointestinal) sensation and bowel motility by stimulating the somatic nervous system and vagus nerve.

Whereas acupuncture has demonstrated significant improvements in IBS symptoms in some IBS patients, no difference was found in the global outcome measurements between other IBS patients who received real or sham (fake) acupuncture. An overview of the documented trials using acupuncture for IBS found that the evidence regarding the efficacy of this type of intervention was inconclusive. This observation suggests that the reported effect of acupuncture may have been due to the placebo effect.

Herbal Therapy

In traditional Chinese medicine, IBS is considered to be the result of stagnated liver energy and a spleen dysfunction. Hence, the aims of Chinese herbal treatments for IBS are to restore the energy of the liver, and to relieve the suppressed spleen function. There are many Chinese herbal formulations for IBS, such as Tong Yao Fang (containing up to 20 herbal ingredients), which is the essential formula for abdominal pain and diarrhea, and the Tibetan herbal formulation Padma Lax. The efficacy of this type of treatment remains controversial.

Cognitive Behavioral Therapy

In order to apply cognitive behavioral therapy in IBS patients, two assumptions must be accepted: (1) IBS symptoms are acquired (learned) and reflect specific skill deficits in cognitive and behavioral functioning, and (2) teaching and rehearsing skills for modifying maladaptive behaviors and thinking patterns can remediate these deficits, which in turn will relieve the symptoms. Although the efficacy of cognitive behavioral therapy in IBS remains controversial, as is the case for herbal therapies, the common belief is that cognitive behavioral therapy may help patients to cope with their symptoms without necessarily abolishing them.

Psychodynamic Interpersonal Therapy

Psychodynamic interpersonal therapy could lead to significant life changes and to improvements in the patient's emotional state, IBS symptoms, and quality of life. This is achieved by helping the patient to understand how his or her emotional state is related to stress and the link between emotions and bowel symptoms. Moreover, it provides the patient with insights into why symptoms develop in the context of difficulties or changes in key relationships.

Relaxation Training

Relaxation training, such as yoga meditation, biofeedback, and progressive muscle relaxation, has proven beneficial in some IBS patients. However, it is unclear how much of the effect of relaxation training is caused by increased attention from the therapist. This approach can be useful in patients for whom stress is an important factor in triggering IBS symptoms. Moreover, relaxation training can be used as a complementary strategy to other nonmedication measures on bad days.

Psychological Treatment

It is rather difficult to evaluate the role of psychological therapy in the management of IBS. The studies conducted to document its effect do not allow an unequivocal conclusion to be drawn due to the designs of the studies, how patients have been selected, and how the results have been interpreted.

Chapter 6
Treatment Options Involving Medication

Summary

- Medications for irritable bowel syndrome (IBS) are symptoms-based, focusing on the main (i.e., most troubling) symptom for the patient.
- Loperamide, which is an opiate-like medication, is effective against diarrhea.
- Tricyclic antidepressants alter pain perception, but have strong side effects.
- Selective serotonin-reuptake inhibitor antidepressants have global benefits without affecting bowel symptoms.
- Bulking agents, and osmotic and emollient laxatives are effective against constipation.
- Prucalopride, linaclotide, and lubiprostone are three new medications that are effective against constipation and reduce abdominal pain and distention.

Since the cause of IBS is not firmly established, treatment with medications is symptom-based, and focuses on the symptom that troubles the patient the most. Thus, medications designed to ameliorate abdominal pain and/or bloating, diarrhea, and constipation are the most commonly prescribed (Table 6.1).

M. El-Salhy et al., *Understanding and Controlling the Irritable Bowel*, DOI 10.1007/978-3-319-15642-2_6,
© Springer International Publishing Switzerland 2015

TABLE 6.1 Medications available for the treatment of IBS

Name	Dose	Effect	Type
Loperamide	2 mg with each loose stool, to a maximum of 16 mg/day	Reduces diarrhea	Opiate-like
Desipramide	10–150 mg at night	Reduces diarrhea, abdominal distension, and pain	Tricyclic antidepressants
Amitriptyline	10–150 mg at night	Improves well-being without benefit to bowel symptoms	Selective serotonin-reuptake inhibitors
Nortriptyline	10–150 mg at night		
Paroxetine	20–50 mg daily		
Fluoxetine	10–40 mg daily		
Rifaximin	400–550 mg three times daily for 7–10 days	Total improvement of symptoms, especially bloating and distension	Antibiotics
Neomycin	1 g daily for 10 days		
Metronidazole	400 mg twice daily for 15 days		

Psyllium	2.5–30 g daily in divided doses	Improves constipation	Bulking agents
Ispaghula	3.5 g from one to three times daily		
Polyethylene glycol	17 g in 237 ml of solution daily	Improves constipation	Osmotic laxative
Mineral oil	5–10 cm^3 daily	Improves constipation	Emollient laxative
Prucalopride	1–2 mg daily	Improves constipation, reduces abdominal pain and distension	Serotonin-hormone-like (agonist)
Linaclotide	290 µg daily	Improves constipation, reduces abdominal pain and distension	Guanylin-hormone-like (agonist)
Lubiprostone	24 µg twice daily	Improves constipation, reduces abdominal pain and distension	Fatty acid derivative, which enhances large-bowel fluid secretion
Hyoscyamine sulfate	0.125 mg up to four times daily	Limited proven efficacy	Antispasmodic
Dicyclomine	10–20 mg from two to four times daily		

Serotonin

Serotonin is an important hormone in the gastrointestinal tract, and an abnormality in it is believed to play an important role in the development of IBS. Hence, several medications used to treat IBS exert their effects by affecting this hormone. Serotonin is produced in two places in the human body: the gastrointestinal tract and the brain. About 90 % of our serotonin is produced in the gastrointestinal tract, about 5 % in the brain; 3–5 % of the serotonin secreted from the bowel is attached to the platelets that circulate in the blood. Serotonin-secreting endocrine cells occurs in several segments of the gastrointestinal tract, namely the stomach, and the small and large bowels. Serotonin-secreting cells are numerous and are the most abundant endocrine cell type in the gastrointestinal tract. Serotonin activates the sensory nerves in the nerve component of the NES (i.e., the enteric nervous system) within the gastrointestinal tract wall, which convey sensation from the gastrointestinal tract to the central nervous system. It also stimulates the nerve cells within the walls of the gastrointestinal tract that initiate the peristaltic reflexes that propel food from the mouth (undigested) to the anus (fecal remains).

Diarrhea in IBS patients can be treated with loperamide or diphenoxylate. Loperamide is an opiate-like (agonist) that does not cross the blood–brain barrier (i.e., it does not reach the brain) and exerts morphine-like effects. It is widely used in clinical practice because it is effective for urgent loose stools, and it is safe, well tolerated, and inexpensive. Loperamide stimulates the absorption of water and electrolytes, inhibits the secretion of water, and slows bowel movements. However, it is not effective for abdominal pain.

Tricyclic antidepressants are used to treat IBS patients, and especially those with diarrhea as the predominant symptom. These medications increase the levels of serotonin by inhibiting its destruction. They alter pain perception in addition to their antidepressant or antianxiety effects. However, tricyclic antidepressants reportedly cause the following side effects in more than one-third of patients: dry mouth, constipation, fatigue, and drowsiness.

Treatment with selective serotonin-reuptake inhibitor antidepressants, which also increase the concentration of serotonin, has been shown to lead to a significant improvement in health-related quality of life in patients with chronic or treatment-resistant IBS. These medications confer global benefits without significant changes in bowel symptoms or pain, and are better tolerated by patients than tricyclic antidepressants.

Antibiotics are used in the treatment of IBS with global relief of IBS symptoms and bloating. However, these good effects have a short duration (up to 3 months). The idea behind using antibiotics in the treatment of IBS is based on the assumption that IBS symptoms could be caused by small-bowel bacterial overgrowth. Another explanation for the beneficial effect of antibiotics is that they kill the large-bowel bacteria and enable potential recolonization with more beneficial bacteria.

Soluble fiber and bulking agents are the most frequently used first-line treatment for constipation. These agents include psyllium, methylcellulose, and calcium polycarbophil. Bulking agents containing insoluble fiber often have the adverse effects of inducing bloating and flatulence. Psyllium and ispaghula (a derivative of psyllium), which contain mainly soluble fiber, have a good effect on constipation and are free from the side effects of other bulking agents.

Osmotic laxatives such as polyethylene glycol and lactulose are used for constipation in IBS, although lactulose, which belongs to FODMAPs, is itself associated with bloating and abdominal pain and is not suitable for long-term use. Stimulant laxatives such as bisacodyl and senna are effective but are associated with abdominal cramping, electrolyte depletion, and diarrhea, and consequently should not be used for long periods.

Three new medications against constipation have recently been introduced onto the market: prucalopride, linaclotide, and lubiprostone. Although these medications are effective and have few side effects, they are expensive.

Prucalopride is a serotonin-like chemical (agonist) that mimics the action of serotonin by stimulating gastrointestinal tract motility. It is effective in IBS patients who do not respond to laxatives. Prucalopride is safe in the elderly, who often suffer from cardiovascular diseases. In addition to its effect on constipation so as to normalize bowel habits, it reduces abdominal pain and distension. Several studies have shown that patients suffering from constipation have low gastrointestinal serotonin. Thus, treatment with prucalopride acts not only as a medication, but also to correct a preexisting defect in these patients. Diarrhea, nausea, abdominal pain, and headache are the common side effects of this medication; however, these side effects disappear in most patients after the first 2 days of taking it. Prucalopride is approved for continuous daily use, and the effect of taking it on demand is not known.

Linaclotide, which is a guanylin-hormone-like (agonist), mimics the action of guanylin on the cells lining the large-bowel lumen to increase fluid secretion. Moreover, linaclotide accelerates gastrointestinal motility. It is effective in the treatment of constipation and reduces abdominal pain and distension. The common side effects of this medication are diarrhea, dizziness, abdominal pain and distention, and flatulence. Like prucalopride, linaclotide is approved for continuous daily use, and the effect of taking it on demand is not known.

Lubiprostone is a fatty-acid derivative that causes an increase in the secretion of fluid into the intestines. This fluid softens the stool and speeds up its passage through the large bowel. Lubiprostone is effective against constipation and reduces abdominal pain and distention. The most common side effects are mild diarrhea, nausea, vomiting, headache, dizziness, and abdominal pain and bloating.

Antispasmodics (i.e., muscle-relaxing agents) are used to relieve IBS symptoms. These agents are designed to relax the smooth muscles within the gastrointestinal tract, especially after ingesting food. However, the efficacy of these agents in the treatment of IBS is limited.

Administration of 3 mg of melatonin at bedtime reduces abdominal pain and rectal pain sensitivity. The beneficial effects of melatonin are independent of its action on sleep disturbances or psychological profiles.

Oil extracts from the peppermint plant (*Mentha piperita*, Lamiaceae) are one of the oldest remedies for the treatment of gastrointestinal problems. These extracts are believed to improve IBS symptoms by exerting a relaxing (spasmolytic) effect on the smooth muscles of the gastrointestinal tract. Although treatment with peppermint oil improves IBS symptoms, further studies are needed to clarify several aspects concerning this treatment such as the side effects and the beneficial effects after long-term use.

Chapter 7
There Is a Light at the End of the Tunnel

Summary

- Although irritable bowel syndrome (IBS) is a tortuous disorder and interferes with the patients' daily activities, it does not develop into a serious disease or kill its sufferer.
- There is evidence that IBS can be inherited.
- In mild and moderate IBS, a combination of dietary management, probiotic intake, and regular exercise are sufficient to control the symptoms. This can be supplemented by taking an appropriate medication on bad days.
- In severe IBS, gastrointestinal-directed hypnosis is effective.
- There are effective symptom-based medications for IBS.
- Patient motivation, collaboration, and a will to make lifestyle adjustments are required to control IBS and enable these patients to lead a normal life.
- There has been progress in our understanding and treatment of IBS and in society's attitude toward this condition.
- Intensive research is being carried out all over the world in efforts to improve the lot of IBS sufferers: there is a light at the end of the tunnel.

IBS is a common disorder, but although patients with IBS suffer considerably as a result of this disorder, due to its interfering with their daily activities, they are not at risk of developing a serious disease or dying because of it. Family clustering of IBS, and the findings of twin and genetic studies indicate that IBS can be inherited. Understanding and learning ways of controlling IBS not only help patients to lead a normal life, but also enable them to help their children and closest relatives.

IBS symptoms are intermittent, and their frequency and severity can vary considerably in the same person over time. In most IBS patients, combining dietary management, probiotic intake, and regular exercise is sufficient to control their symptoms. While extra medication and/or extra exercise will help patients with mild or moderate forms of IBS to get through particularly bad days, this approach alone is not enough for patients with the severe form of IBS—gastrointestinal-directed hypnosis has proven to be effective in those patients.

There are effective medications for the treatment of IBS symptoms such as diarrhea, constipation, and abdominal pain, and intensive research activities are ongoing all around the world to find or develop more.

There is no miracle treatment for IBS. In order to control IBS and lead a normal life, patients must be motivated, cooperate with their healthcare providers, and be willing to make lifestyle adjustments. In doing so, we have seen patients with long sick-leave return to work and students who have dropped out of their studies return to the school bench. We have also seen patients regaining the energy and will to restore broken relationships or to break up nonfunctioning relationships.

Clinical experience shows that patients with IBS whose bowel symptoms are improved also experience improvements in other IBS-associated symptoms (see Chap. 1) such as depression, headache, insomnia, fatigue, and muscle pain. We have no explanation for such improvements.

There is extensive IBS research being conducted all around the world, and every day we gain more knowledge about its cause and how best to treat it. Moreover, societal attitudes toward IBS are changing, and healthcare providers, gastroenterology societies, and gastroenterology patient organizations in several countries are now taking both IBS itself and IBS patients seriously. In other words, there is a light at the end of the tunnel.

Appendices

Appendix A

Gastroscopy

The Gastroscope

The gastroscope is an approximately 1-m-long, thin flexible rubber tube (about 10 mm in diameter), at the top of which there is a source for illumination, a camera, and holes for taking tissue samples, suctioning, air insufflation (blowing air into the esophagus, stomach, and proximal small bowel lumen to be able to see these gastrointestinal segments clearly), and cleaning the camera lens. At the other end of the gastroscope there is a device that is controlled by the examining doctor that enables bending of the top of the gastroscope to different angles (Fig. 1). The gastroscope is attached to several machines that allow the performance of various functions during the procedure (i.e., related to diagnosis, surveillance, and therapy).

How Gastroscopy Is Done

Gastroscopy is usually performed after an overnight fast, although a 4- to 6-h fast seems to be sufficient. Local anesthesia is administered to the patient's throat, and a plastic ring is placed inside mouth around the teeth to protect

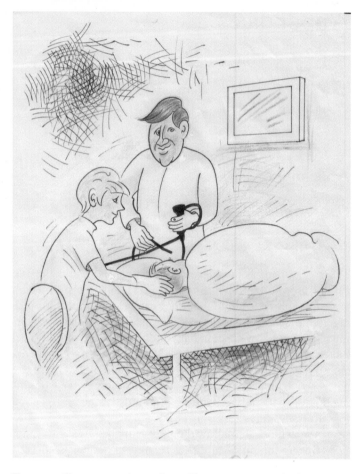

FIGURE 1 Gastroscopy is conducted by a gastroenterologist assisted by a nurse. This procedure is usually rapid and is not painful, but can be unpleasant

both the patient's teeth and the gastroscope. The examination is done with the patient lying on the left side, and is performed by a gastroenterologist, who is assisted by a nurse. It typically takes 5–15 min and is not painful, but can be uncomfortable. Complications associated with this examination are extremely rare. Patients can suffer from a sore throat after the examination, but this normalizes rapidly (after 12–24 h). Sedation is necessary in patients with a strong vomiting reflex, and in a few cases general anesthesia has to be used.

The Purpose of Gastroscopy

Gastroscopy can be used to examine the esophagus, stomach, and the proximal (first) part of the small bowel. During this procedure, small superficial tissue samples can be taken (biopsies) for later examination under a microscope (Fig. 2).

What Gastroscopy Can Identify

Gastroscopy can reveal ulceration, inflammation, tumors, or polyps. Moreover, as mentioned above, tissue samples can be taken from the small bowel for further microscopic examination for the diagnosis of celiac disease.

Appendix B

Colonoscopy

The Colonoscope

The colonoscope is a flexible rubber tube that is slightly longer and thicker than a gastroscope (about 1.5 m long with a diameter of about 13 mm). Like the gastroscope, the top of the colonoscope is provided with a source for illumination, a camera, and holes for taking tissue samples, suctioning, air insufflation, and cleaning the camera lens. The other end of the colonoscope possesses the same devices as the gastroscope.

How Colonoscopy Is Done

Bowel cleansing is required before colonoscopy. This is achieved by ingesting a solution either dissolved in water or in concentrated form 1 day before the examination. If the

FIGURE 2 Photographs of (a) the esophagus, (b) the stomach, and (c) the duodenum (the first part of the small intestine) as seen through a gastroscope. The esophagus is a straight smooth tube, the stomach has a thick trabeculated wall, and the duodenum has a typical villous structure, which can be seen at the bottom of the picture

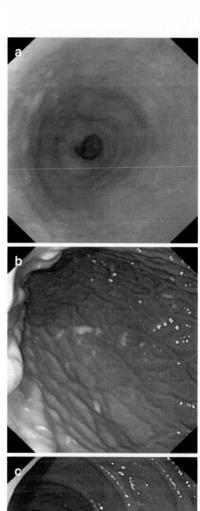

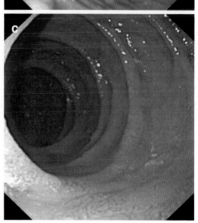

concentrated solution is taken, a large quantity (e.g., 4 l) of liquid should also be taken (e.g., water, tea, juices, or soup). This triggers diarrhea, and the bowel is considered clean when the feces comprise only colored liquid. The patient may eat a light breakfast on the day of the examination. Before the examination, the patient usually receives an analgesic (pain-killer, morphine-like) medication, relaxants (benzodi-azepines), and medication against the nausea that can be caused by the analgesic (Fig. 3).

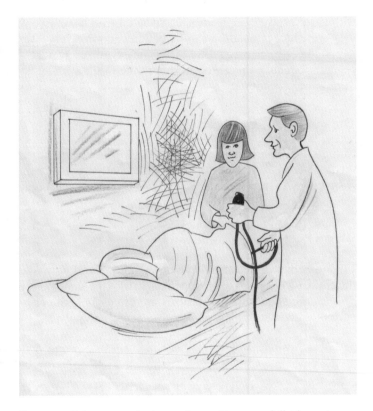

FIGURE 3 Colonoscopy is also performed by a specialist in gastroenterology assisted by a nurse. A colonoscopy can be painful and so patients usually receive sedation, and it normally takes 20–30 min

The patient lies on the left side initially, but the position can be changed during the examination if required. The examination is performed by a gastroenterologist assisted by a nurse, and usually takes between 20 and 30 min, but it can take less or more time depending on the spatial arrangement of the large bowel. During the examination insufflation is a crucial aspect of the colonoscopy procedure, for inflating the bowel to allow its visualization. Carbon dioxide (CO_2) is usually used instead of air. CO_2 absorbed quicker than air, and consequently disappears from the bowel faster than air. As with gastroscopy, complications associated with colonoscopy are rare. The examination can be painful, and in a few cases general anesthesia is required. After the examination, a transient abdominal pain can occur due to the insufflation of air during the procedure.

The Purpose of Colonoscopy

Colonoscopy can be used to examine all of the segments of the large bowel and the distal part of the small bowel. As with gastroscopy, tissue samples can be taken for later microscopic examination (Fig. 4).

What Colonoscopy Can Identify

Colonoscopy can detect inflammation, tumors, and polyps in the entire large bowel and in the distal part of the small bowel. This examination in IBS patients is used to exclude the presence of inflammatory bowel diseases, cancer, and polyps.

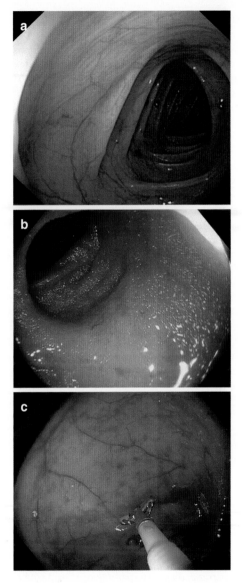

FIGURE 4 The appearance of (**a**) the colon and (**b**) the ileum (the last part of the small intestine) as seen through a colonoscope. (**c**) The biopsy forceps can be seen, which are used to remove small samples of tissue for further analysis (if required)

References

The data presented in this book are based on the clinical experience of the authors, their research, and recently published scientific articles. A short list of the main references is given below:

1. El-Salhy M. Irritable bowel syndrome: diagnosis and pathogenesis. World J Gastroenterol. 2012;18:5151–63.
2. El-Salhy M, Gilja OH, Gundersen D, Hatlebakk JG, Hausken T. Interaction between ingested nutrients and gut endocrine cells in patients with irritable bowel syndrome (Review). Int J Mol Med. 2014;34:363–71.
3. El-Salhy M, Gundersen D, Gilja OH, Hatlebakk JG, Hausken T. Is irritable bowel syndrome an organic disorder? World J Gastroenterol. 2014;2:384–400.
4. El-Salhy M, Hatlebakk JG, Gilja OH, Hausken T. Irritable bowel syndrome: recent developments in diagnosis, pathophysiology, and treatment. Expert Rev Gastroenterol Hepatol. 2014;8:435–43.
5. El-Salhy M, Ostgaard H, Gundersen D, Hatlebakk JG, Hausken T. The role of diet in the pathogenesis and management of irritable bowel syndrome (Review). Int J Mol Med. 2012;29:723–31.
6. El-Salhy M, Seim I, Chopin L, Gundersen D, Hatlebakk JG, Hausken T. Irritable bowel syndrome: the role of gut neuroendocrine peptides. Front Biosci (Elite Ed). 2012;4:2783–800.
7. Mazzawi T, Hausken T, Gundersen D, El-Salhy M. Effects of dietary guidance on the symptoms, quality of life and habitual dietary intake of patients with irritable bowel syndrome. Mol Med Rep. 2013;8:845–52.
8. Ostgaard H, Hausken T, Gundersen D, El-Salhy M. Diet and effects of diet management on quality of life and symptoms in patients with irritable bowel syndrome. Mol Med Rep. 2012;5:1382–90.
9. Lee YJ, Park KS. Irritable bowel syndrome: emerging paradigm in pathophysiology. World J Gastroenterol. 2014;20:2456–69.
10. Soares RL. Irritable bowel syndrome: a clinical review. World J Gastroenterol. 2014;20:12144–60.
11. El-Salhy M, Gundersen D, Hatlebakk JG, Hausken T. Irritable bowel syndrome: diagnosis, pathogenesis and treatment options. New York: Nova Science Publishers, Inc.; 2012.

Index

M. El-Salhy et al., *Understanding and Controlling the Irritable*   83
Bowel, DOI 10.1007/978-3-319-15642-2,
© Springer International Publishing Switzerland 2015

Printed by Printforce, the Netherlands